Salute to

Philadelphia

VA

Medical Center

*

Thank You!

Reverend Mike Wanner

Table of Contents

Dedication

This book is dedicated to all those who have served to defend the United States of America and their families who have served also, by missing them during their service and some forever. These valiant citizens have given freely in the pursuit of the noble goals specified in the Declaration of Independence and the Constitution of The United States and all the amendments thereto.

I give special recognition to those who have been killed in the service of our country. The citizens now and future citizens of the United States of America will be forever in their debt. May all who have served and their families be blessed in the now and the forever AND SO IT IS!

Special recognition goes also to those injured in the service of our country. The United States of America will be forever in their debt. The injured warriors of our nation have performed well a duty and this writing is offered to help mitigate some of the emotional turmoil that may still reside within those valiant ones. May each of them and their families be blessed in all ways AND SO IT IS!

It is the intent of this work to help Veterans to reclaim their power after their military service is complete.

May All who Read this book be Blessed AND SO IT IS!

Reverend Mike Wanner

Acknowledgements

I would like to acknowledge the support of the following beings:

Ceil Nuyianes is an Earth Angel who started as a student of mine in Reiki and developed into a friend whose book industry expertise helped guide me in many ways.

Mary E Jay who has been an inspiration.

Nancy Russell who was my Integrated Energy Therapy Master Instructor who introduced me to Angel Ariel and the methodology of Heartlinking with the Angels to facilitate the clearing of stuffed emotions and cellular memory.

Stevan Thayer who was my Integrated Energy Therapy Master Instructor Trainer who taught me how to teach others - How to Heal with The Energy of Angels.

My Reiki Masters Rita Hildenbrandt, Hannelore Goodwin, Gary Jirauch, Tom Rigler, Patrick Zigler, Hiroshi Doi, Chiyoko Yamaguchi, Tadao Yamaguchi and especially the founder of Komyo Kai Reiki Reverend Hyakuten Inamoto.

Reverend Ethel Lomardi who taught me the healing power of viewing people as pure light.

Archangels Michael - the Protector, Gabriel - the Communicator, Raphael- the Healer and the legions of Angels that help the healing process for all.

Introduction

This book started as a kind of thank you card to the practitioners and staff that have cared for me during my visits to the VA.

The news reports daily talk about all that is wrong with the VA and it does bother me to hear that some have been underserved. I also know that there is great good going on within the VA. Failure to recognize the good can stifle the spirit of those that are doing the good and create a situation that does not elevate performance for the employees, the administration or the veterans.

The responsibility for assisting Veterans is assigned to the VA but I think that the responsibility needs to be spread around a lot.

So I will structure this as a Thank You that I and all Philadelphia VA Medical Center visitors can use PLUS.

I know that it could be expensive for People to buy this book for that purpose so I would encourage others to send their own Thank You Cards. If you want to piggyback on this project, you might want to write, I agree with Mike – Philadelphia VAMC is EXCELLENT or recognize the VAMC in your community.

Chapter 1 - Thank You

If your name or department appears on the name line below and is signed by me or another veteran below that then you are one of the excellent people or teams that the signer has had the pleasure to meet personally and salutes now for your part in the care received. You have also been part of the representation of the Philadelphia VA Medical Center upon which is based the opinion of consistently excellent effort.

I Salute

Name/Dept. _____

Many thanks to you and all your unnamed colleagues for your professional diagnosis, analysis and service to me and many other veterans.

_____

Date_____

Chapter 2 - What Is This Book About?

As a former aircraft mechanic and maintenance workload controller and laboratory scheduler in the USAF, I understand about scheduling. After returning to civilian life, my skills moved me up with my former employer (Sears) to an efficiency expert type of position so I see things a little differently than the casual observer.

At the Philadelphia VA Medical Center, I see a lot of wonderful people working very hard to help the veterans with the traditional care giving modalities and the work they do is outstanding. My experience is limited to those departments that I actually visited but it is indicative of the great good that is happening.

 I do want everyone at the Philadelphia VAMC to know that your diligence is recognized and appreciated and that the effort to help veterans should not be yours alone.

I hope that this little book can help share some ideas that can help veterans by having others help them get ready to receive your professional excellence.

Chapter 3 - Excellent in Philadelphia

I want to share the excellence of my experience but I have not used every part of the system. I share my experience as it is and hope that it helps to recognize some hard working folks. Here is what I liked:

General Practitioner

My primary consult and assignment was with Dr. G, a general practitioner at the Victor J. Saracini Outpatient Clinic in Horsham, PA. Dr. G was very methodical in going over my medical history and records.

His demeanor and information were very helpful to my understanding of what the clinic and the hospital have to offer and what they do not.

I was very pleased with the process of the VA system as the patient care is put first and the bureaucracy is minimal. Dr. G has proven over time to be consistently excellent in his job that insures that all care is integrated and coordinated. I am most grateful for his excellence.

The nurses and support staff at the Saracini clinic seem to be consistently awesome but one nurse absolutely astounded me. She calls herself Lovey and does very well and without any discomfort what nobody else seems to be able to do.

The needle access area in the crease between my forearm and upper arm has no visible veins to be tapped. The American Red Cross won't even take my blood because it is too hard to get.

Most blood drawers use my hand as the veins are easy to find and access. Lovey goes in to the crease and gets blood without any discomfort or a second attempt. WOW.

Rheumatology

My first clinical stop in Philadelphia was Rheumatology and I was very happy with the transition of my therapy. Doctor O. was my primary Rheumatologist and her supervisor was a legend in the specialty – Dr. P.

The care received was precise and methodical and the analysis of my status was consistently diligent. It was a delight to see the process of both the younger doctor and the supervisor as they deliberately explored every conceivable option and brought in others for consultation. Dr. O was replaced with Dr. K and then Dr. G with consistent diligent excellence.

The care went well and the cooperation level with surgical teams was very well done. Others in the department who are worthy of an excellent rating are Carmen from the reception desk and Gilda the nurse.

After four years of treatment, everything remains excellent. There was a bit of a miracle this year as I transitioned after my IV medication interruption for surgery procedures. I was on an Intravenous Therapy called Remaicade which suppressed my immune system and was stopped a month before foot surgery on five toes.

The five toes surgery took a very long time for the healing process to complete. I was on and off antibiotics four times before the wound healing cleared.

When podiatry finally cleared me, I went back to Rheumatology and Dr. G was happy to see that I had not deteriorated like they would have expected from previous patterns. He called in Dr. P and she was all smiles. She called in another doctor and they were all happy about my Rheumatology progress.

A new medication was ordered that is much less powerful and less risky. I was smiling too. Thank you very much.

Short Procedure Unit

My second clinical stop in Philadelphia was the Short Procedure Unit. This was where I received the Intravenous infusion every eight weeks.

The short procedure unit is a busy place filled with patients coming and going all day long. I got to know the staff over four years of getting IVs.

The good humor, good nature, professionalism and kindness of each team member is very clear. Smiling under pressure can require a lot of discipline and these delightful staff members embody the pinnacle level of their craft. Well done all.

Operating Room

While the operating room is not my favorite place, I appreciated the service very much. From the Short Procedure Unit to the transport team to the prep room to the Operating Room to the surgery itself to the Post OP to the transport team return and back to Short Procedure Unit, there was a consistent awareness of potential anxiety and the mitigation thereof.

Kindness was consistent throughout the experience and it really helped. Thank you very much.

Podiatry

My podiatry experience was long and involved but consistently excellent throughout. The teamwork in the department was quite awesome. I don't think that I have ever seen a more interactive group of professionals.

The team integration was consistently inspiring and just plain fun. How can such a serious thing be fun? It starts with the demeanor of lightheartedness and professionalism and continues with methodical precision.

If anybody needs foot surgery or care, Philly VAMC Podiatry gets my vote of Excellence. There was a time where my right toes looked like five rows of ground meat but now they look like toes again. Thanks so much.

A list of these great doctors would require the whole alphabet and I would run the risk of missing one so my gratitude is to the whole department which runs like a well maintained Swiss clock from reception to assistants to students to the doctors and fabulous good natured supervisors who really honor the gifts of fellow team members at all levels.

Blood Drawing

You never know what to expect when you enter the waiting room as they serve a lot of people and if you are a minute earlier or later, your wait can be radically different.

What I really like is the temperament of the staff as they just grin and bear the unpredictable workload as it arrives. They don't seem to get flustered or reckless under pressure. They just perform excellent professional deliberate service.

The really nice part is that they are consistently present with the client they are working with and their focus is on the one they are serving and nothing else.

The physical space of the department has been physically rehabbed and the flow and the ambience have been enhanced. Thank you very much.

XRAY

The XRAY department reception is a busy place. There are a lot of different types of XRAY services being provided.

While the workload is intermittent depending on many factors, the clerical staff and professional technicians seem to integrate about as flawlessly as you could expect at a medical facility.

Everybody throughout the department seems to be giving a maximum collective effort of excellence and productivity. They are thoughtful, respectful and fired up with a wanting to serve well. Thanks.

Pharmacy

Pharmacy seems to be the busiest department of the hospital. I get all my scheduled medications accurately filled every single time. If there is a question, they are very direct with the right answer the first time. Thank you very much.

Sleep Center

I have had Sleep Apnea for many years before coming to the VA Hospital and have been very pleased with the continued support that the VA has performed. There was an upgrade in the machine they wanted me to use so they can continue to monitor and tweak my pressures.

Interesting enough is that the vendor changes they have made had no negative consequences as the employees from one vendor seem to move over to the new vendor.

Dermatology

I was referred to dermatology for a few concerns and was very happy with each visit. I saw a number of practitioners and the interactions were flawless.

Emergency Room

I only made a couple of trips to the Emergency Room and one seemed very fast and the other took a while. As I was writing, my guidance kicked in and suggested that the VA should not be held to a higher standard than every other Emergency Room so I soon realized that even what I thought of as slow was much better than most other times I went to or took someone to a community ER.

The time that was quick had me on an IV before the test results came back. The doctor even said after looking at me that I would be staying before the tests were even ordered.

Urology

One of the trips to the ER had me ending up with a Urology consult that left me with a treatment plan that did not thrill me. A CAT scan in a few weeks to see if I had kidney stones and a surgery date many weeks later.

I consulted with an outside doctor because I had blood in my urine and the feeling was that I might do well to consider using my private insurance to move up the surgery. I kept the CAT scan appointment and sought an earlier surgery date with a private hospital and then cancelled the VA surgery date while keeping everybody in the loop of my intentions and motivations.

The private hospital did not overwhelm me with diligence. The first surgery date was put off because of a technicality that was not handled well in the pre-admission protocol.

So we had a new surgery date and they went in to take care of the stones in a way that did not thrill me. The earlier delay caused another delay because the stones had moved during this time and they were not permissioned to go where the stones were so they exited.

So we had a new surgery date and they went in again to take care of the stones in a way that did not thrill me. This time (the third scheduled) they were successful.

The delays caused the surgery to be much later than the VA had originally scheduled. The two delays had also caused two procedures instead of one.

My family traveled in from out of state to take care of me for the original procedure that was cancelled at the last minute. And again my family travelled in to take care of me for the second time when the stone wasn't removed because it had moved. And my family travelled in for a third time to take care of me when the stone was actually removed.

So when the dust settled, my experience had me gladly coming back to the VA with a whole new appreciation for the simplicity and speed of the VA sstem.

Computer Systems

The efficiency of the hospital is largely dependent on the flow of information for appointments, Labs, X-rays, testing and specialty appointments etc. As an observer, I see excellence again and I especially like the reminder list of appointments and the medication list.

The appointment list keeps everybody aware of the timelines for the patient. Practitioners have been diligent when I have had multiple appointments in the same day so that if at all possible, they help me to finish in time to be timely for my next appointment. I suspect but don't know that they would also be helpful to notify any departments that would be impacted if it was not possible.

The medication list is helpful to remember what one needs to take and also as a tool in an emergency. The medication list is a big part of patient history and my ambulance career tells me clearly how important that is.

I wonder whether it would be possible (Maybe not because of privacy) for the list to include a line of the patient's diagnosis so that it would turn in to a type of easily portable Medical History record that the patient could carry with them for any emergency they might have anywhere.

We all know that a good medical history can save a life. Also for consideration, would be a notice of some sort that says to the patient that it would be a good idea to keep your medication record with you in case of emergency.

Chapter 4 - Too Much Blame on The VA

I feel very deliberately that there is too much blame placed on the VA which is charged with picking up the pieces of many tragedies.

I would encourage all involved with the military to establish a debriefing discharge protocol for every branch of the service. A little time spent in preparation could well be basic training for reintegration to the civilian world.

Debriefing is done in critical incidents because a lot can be learned and that can avoid the same problems being created again in similar scenarios. We know that a lot of veterans do not integrate back to civilian life as well as we might like.

A little diligence done in the discharge process can pay huge dividends in quality of life for veterans and expense avoidance for the nation.

Chapter 5 - Possibilities For Change At The VA Medical Centers

I wrote a whole book called *Trauma Healing Options For VA Hospitals: Help For Veterans to Own Their Healing And Their Future.* This book is part of my Veterans Healing six pack and is available free on kindle at specific times. Everybody can join the notification list of when the books are free at http://VeteransHealing.withRevMike.com .

I well understand that the budgets and processes of the VA are established in advance and I find no fault with the absence of my suggestions. I also know that somebody has to be bold enough to ask others to think outside the box and I am respectfully doing that by asking VA staff to download that book when it is free and use it for a reference as you plan the participation of your department in future veteran healing strategies.

Change takes time, so please do not give up if there is no rapid acceptance of your ideas that grow out of my suggestions. Patience is still a virtue and carrying the banner of things that can work will offer you a level of personal peace and stress reduction.

Chapter 6 - Churches and Veteran Service Organizations Can Help

Just like part of the VA's burden should be shifted to the military, part of it can be shared by churches and Veteran Service Organizations that are willing to help.

I wrote a little book called *Tea for Veterans: Welcome One Home* which lays out many possibilities. This book is part of my Veterans Healing six pack and is available free on kindle at specific times. Everybody can join the notification list of when the books are free at http://VeteransHealing.withRevMike.com

The idea is simple enough. Churches and Veteran Service organization can team up to offer a safe space to welcome veterans home. They put it on their community calendars and cross promote it so veterans learn about the availability.

Chapter 7 - Veterans Can Help

Veterans are very resourceful and they can do a lot for each other. This is mentioned in detail in the Trauma Healing Options for VA Hospitals Book.

I have also created a series of DIY books Called Trauma Healing Action Steps for Veterans. Each book focus is different and there is a book focused on Help to Get Started, Empowerment, Forgiveness and Thought freedom.

The books are part of my Veterans Healing six pack and they are available free on kindle at specific times. Everybody can join the notification list of when the books are free at http://VeteransHealing.withRevMike.com

The full titles are:

- Trauma Healing Action Steps for Veterans: Help To Start Healing
- Trauma Healing Action Steps for Veterans: Empowerment
- Trauma Healing Action Steps for Veterans: Forgiveness

- Trauma Healing Action Steps for Veterans: Thought Freedom.

No Kindle is required to download the books. Amazon.com has a free application that offers "Kindle for PC" software and "Kindle for Mac" software where you can download the free appropriate application and then download the books when they are offered.

Chapter 8 - Reiki Practitioners Can Help

In my Veterans Healing books, I talk a lot about Reiki modalities that could be used to help veterans. I am taking the time here to invite practitioners of Reiki to get creative and invite themselves to the party.

Veterans may well be too timid to bring their needs to your attention. Veterans Hospitals may be a long time in getting authorization to fund any kind of Reiki program.

I invite Reiki Practitioner to reach out to the Veteran Service Organizations and try to create win-win situations where there is benefit to all.

If you are a Reiki Master and you need a place to hold a class, you could approach a Veteran Service Organization (American Legion, Veterans of Foreign Wars, Disabled American Veterans) and suggest they host your class in exchange for free sessions by your students for veterans.

Creativity can benefit all.

Chapter 9 - Integrated Energy Therapy® Practitioners Can Help

I write a lot about Integrated Energy Therapy® helping veterans. I now invite practitioners of IET to get creative and invite themselves to the veteran's community.

Veterans may well be too withdrawn to bring their needs to your attention. Veterans Hospitals will likely be a long time in getting authorization to fund any kind of IET program.

I invite you to reach out to the Veteran Service Organizations and try to create win-win situations where there is benefit to all.

If you are a Master Instructor and you need a place to hold a class, you could approach a Veteran Service Organization (American Legion, Veterans of Foreign Wars, Disabled American Veterans) and suggest they host your class in exchange for free sessions by your students for veterans.

A major capability of IET is help with stuffed emotions and many veterans need that help. Creativity can benefit all.

Chapter 10 - Energy Medicine

An emerging field of study called energy medicine is aligned with the spiritual energy modalities that have been so successful for many years.

I would encourage further development of a discussion on energy medicine throughout the VA Medical community.

The beauty of energy medicine is that much of it can be done by the patients themselves or their families or bodywork practitioners.

A number of the techniques can be investigated to provide personal experiences for veterans that can help them know that they can achieve a new normal that is aligned with them being at peace internally.

I have included some of these systems as separate chapters in my Trauma Healing Options for VA Hospitals book so you can consider them individually.

There is much more to be researched. I share only that which I know and can talk about.

Chapter 11 - Unchain the Healing Potential

This can be a great time of expansion in the healing services for all citizens of all nations if we will but begin to expand the potentials of existing systems and encourage emotional breakthroughs at the level of each care receiver.

Emotional Health has changed over the years and this is especially true for those who have experienced the hyper-stimulation of military service. While these times are difficult, there is great opportunity to learn as we go.

Let us all be open to the Divine Help that is always available when we shut out the earthly world and tune in to messages from God AND SO IT IS.

Chapter 12 - All Things Considered

I know that this writing has helped to recognize some of the great people at the Philly VAMC. Many others who work there are also worthy of recognition but I don't know them.

The press seems to never have substantial positive comments to say about the VA. This is unfortunate because a lot of good already exists.

I encourage others to notice the good that is and recognize everybody at the VA everywhere who is trying so hard to help the Veterans. It is important that the consumers (the veterans) speak up in a way that is positive and offers guidance.

It is easy to say that we need an interactive system where providers and veterans have supporters who have the ability to share ideas that can bear fruit for all. I know that will not be easy to do but I float it out there as a possible goal.

May God Bless everybody who is treated by, works in, supports, supplies and interacts with the VA Medical System AND SO IT IS! Thank You God.

ReverendMikeWanner.com
Resources List

Distant Healing Sessions –

Physical Healing
http://LetMeHelpYouHeal.withMike.com

Angel Healing
http://AngelHealing.withmike.com/

Books by Rev. Mike at www.Amazon.com–

Veterans Healing Six Pack:
1. *Trauma Healing options for VA Hospitals: Help for Veterans to Own Their Healing and their future.*
2. *Trauma Healing Action Steps for Veterans: Help to Start Healing*
3. *Trauma Healing Action Steps for Veterans: Empowerment*
4. *Trauma Healing Action Steps for Veterans: Forgiveness*
5. *Trauma Healing Action Steps for Veterans: Thought Freedom*
6. *Tea For Veterans; Welcome One Home*

Angel Raphael Speaks Volume One: Take Courage! God Has Healing in Store for You

Angel Raphael Speaks Volume Two: Take Courage! God Has Healing in Store for You

Reiki Journaling from Japan

Reiki Is Alive: God's Great Gift

Four Parts to Healing

Distant Healing: We Are All Connected

Stress Release Energy Work: How To Cope

Group Consciousness: I Asked The Wind to Blow

The PTSD Project: Turn Pain To Power

Free Resources

Learn to dump fear at
http://TheGreatAmericanFearDump.withMike.com

Spiritually Prepare for Surgery
http://PrepareForSurgery.withRevMike.com

Angel Scribe messages at
http://www.SpiritualComfortCare.com

Law of Attraction Expert column at
http://www.ReverendMikeWanner.com

Stress Release at
http://www.StressReleaseCoach.com

Angel Raphael Speaks through Rev. Mike Wanner. I have channeled multiple message sets and they all have to be polished to smooth out my errors and negotiate some words that may be too easily misunderstood. Grammar is not polished as it is too easy to miss the subtlety of the energy flow. To find out the availability of messages and latest updates go to
http://www.spiritualcomfortcare.com/angel-raphael-speaks/

Also "Tell Mike your concerns – If he and I agree there is a broader need, messages may follow. Citizens of all nations invited as long as your write in English. Do not expect him to answer as he is very busy already listening to us." E-mail Mike at mikewann@voicenet.com.

May All Who Read This Be Blessed Reverend Mike Wanner

Join the Veterans Healing FREE Kindle Book Notification List at http://VeteransHealing.withRevMike.com

Private Channeling

Angel Raphael Speaks is a series of free messages that are channeled through Reverend Mike Wanner for the highest good and Highest Healing of all concerned.

Many questions arise about Reverend Mike doing private channeling and he does help with that at his site
http://AngelHealing.withMike.com

Reverend Mike is available world-wide as a psychic channel, emotional release facilitator, spiritual energy practitioner & teacher, and public speaker.

He looks forward to meeting you soon! Email -
mikewann@voicenet.com 215-342-1270
http://AngelHealing.withMike.com

PRIVATE SPIRITUAL READINGS/channelings or Spiritual Healing Sessions: Telephone or in person

Rev. Mike is available for private, one-on-one intuitive sessions with you, his Guide Family, and your Guides. He helps by offering clarity on emotional situations about your life, your purpose, your spirituality, and the release of stuffed emotions and cellular memory.

Connect to the love of your Guides today! Contact Rev. Mike for an appointment soon.

Click on this link to go to the page –
http://AngelHealing.withMike.com

Sessions available:

Spiritual Readings
Angel Channeling
Distant Reiki Healing
Distant Clearing of Stuffed Emotions
Distant Clearing of Cellular Memory
Distant Clearing of Energy Blockages
Distant Clearing of the Chakras
Mastermind dowsing responses to yes/no direction finding questions.
Customized needs

Rev. Mike is a facilitator of healing. He brings you and the Divine together so that you can align with the Divine and have a great time and a great life. All healing is between you and God, as it should be. Go ahead and start without Rev. Mike. Visit his prayer site http://www.Create-A-Prayer.com. Take the first step NOW.

Rev. Michael Wanner

Rev. Michael Wanner started his metaphysical and ministerial studies with Reiki in 1993 and has studied seven styles of Reiki in the U.S., Japan, Canada, Denmark and Australia. He is certified to teach. He became certified to teach Integrated Energy Therapy in 1999 and co-taught the first IET class of the new Millennium. Mike began dowsing in 2001.

Ordained as a Metaphysical Minister of the International Metaphysical Ministry and an Interfaith Minister of the Circle of Miracles Ministry, Rev. Mike practices and teaches spiritual energy therapies in the Philadelphia Area.

Rev. Mike holds ministerial degrees from the University of Metaphysics and the University of Sedona. He is a Pastoral Care Associate of Aria – Frankford Hospital. He taught at the National Academy of Massage Therapy and Health Sciences.

Rev. Mike was a faculty member of the Medical Mission Sister's Center for Human Integration's School of Integrated Body/Mind Therapies in Fox Chase, Philadelphia, PA for twelve years.

Rev. Mike is licensed by the teaching of Intuitional Metaphysics to practice Spiritual Healing and Scientific Prayer. Mike is also a Prayer therapist.

Rev. Mike was elected in 2007 to the status of "Fellow of the American Institute of Stress."

In 2008, Rev. Mike became a practitioner of Coincidental Recognition as he incorporated the CoRe system in to his spiritual healing practice.

In 2009, Rev. Mike trademarked a new healing process called Quantum Quatro! Subtle Energy System Support®.

In 2011, Rev. Mike joined the outreach program known as the Health Advantage Group.

In 2012. Rev. Mike became a Certified Professional Coach by The Master Coaching Academy and Joined The Personal Empowerment Group .

Prior to his metaphysical, ministerial and coaching studies, Rev. Mike worked for Sears Roebuck and Co. while in High School and after graduation until he joined the U. S. Air Force in 1965. He returned to Sears from Vietnam in 1969 and stayed until 1978. His final Sears assignment was as an efficiency expert in Methods - Operational Research and Development.

He volunteered with Burholme Emergency Medical Services from 1969 and is still a Life Member and Board of Directors Member. He started a private ambulance company in 1975 and worked professionally in the field until 2001 when he devoted his full attention to real estate investing, healing and coaching.

www.ReverendMikeWanner.com

www.ingramcontent.com/pod-product-compliance
Lightning Source LLC
Chambersburg PA
CBHW070513290526
45790CB00003B/1216